SLOW COOKER

COOKBOOK

DELICIOUS BUDGET-FRIENDLY RECIPES FOR BEGINNERS

ALEC GREEN

Table of Contents

Simple Chicken Stock

A super basic stock.

Makes about 1.5 litres/2½ pints

1 litre/1¾ pints water

1 cooked or raw chicken carcass, broken into pieces

2 celery sticks, thickly sliced

3 small onions, thickly sliced,

3 carrots, thickly sliced

1 small turnip, quartered

5 garlic cloves

2 bay leaves

½ tsp whole peppercorns

1 tsp dried sage leaves

salt and freshly ground black pepper, to taste

Combine all the ingredients, except the salt and pepper, in the slow cooker. Cover and cook on Low for 6–8 hours. Strain, discarding the meat, vegetables and seasonings. Season to taste with salt and pepper. Refrigerate the stock overnight. Skim the fat from the surface of the stock.

Fresh Chicken Stock

Soups and casseroles are transformed with a good home-made stock, and chicken is the most popular to make and use. Cook this version if you need to make a good stock from scratch.

Makes about 1.5 litres/2½ pints

1 litre/1¾ pints water
1.5 kg/3 lb chicken pieces
2 celery sticks, thickly sliced
3 small onions, thickly sliced,
3 carrots, thickly sliced
1 small turnip, quartered
5 garlic cloves
2 bay leaves
½ tsp whole peppercorns
1 tsp dried sage leaves
salt and freshly ground black pepper, to taste

Combine all the ingredients, except the salt and pepper, in the slow cooker. Cover and cook on Low for 6–8 hours. Strain, discarding the meat, vegetables and seasonings. Season to taste with salt and pepper. Refrigerate the stock overnight. Skim the fat from the surface of the stock.

Rich Chicken Stock

A veal knuckle is added here to make a richer stock. It's an ideal recipe to make when you're entertaining and need a stock that's especially full-flavoured to bring the very best out of the dish you are preparing.

Makes about 3.5 litres/6 pints

3.5 litres/6 pints water
250 ml/8 fl oz dry white wine or water
1 chicken (about 1.5 kg/3 lb), cut into pieces, fat trimmed
1 veal knuckle, cracked (optional)
2 onions, thickly sliced
2 leeks (white parts only), thickly sliced
4 medium carrots, thickly sliced
4 celery sticks, thickly sliced
1 garlic clove, peeled
½ tsp dried basil
½ tsp dried thyme
½ tsp dried tarragon
10 black peppercorns
4 whole cloves
salt and freshly ground black pepper, to taste

Combine all the ingredients, except the salt and pepper, in a 5.5 litre/9½ pint slow cooker. Cover and cook on Low for 6–8 hours.

Strain the stock through a double layer of muslin, discarding the solids. Season to taste with salt and pepper. Refrigerate until chilled. Remove the fat from the surface of the stock.

Turkey Stock

The perfect ending for a Christmas turkey, this stock can be used for Turkey Noodle Soup or as a substitute in recipes calling for chicken stock.

Makes about 3.5 litres/6 pints

3.5 litres/6 pints water
250 ml/8 fl oz dry white wine or water
1 turkey carcass, cut up
2 medium onions, thickly sliced
2 leeks (white parts only), thickly sliced
4 medium carrots, thickly sliced
4 celery sticks, thickly sliced
1 tsp dried thyme
10 black peppercorns
6 sprigs of fresh parsley
salt and freshly ground black pepper, to taste

Combine all the ingredients, except the salt and pepper, in a 5.5 litre/9½ pint slow cooker. Cover and cook on Low for 6–8 hours. Strain the stock through a double layer of muslin, discarding the solids. Season to taste with salt and pepper. Refrigerate until chilled. Remove the fat from the surface of the stock.

Beef Stock

A good beef stock is perfect for meat dishes and soups that require a stronger flavour. Although a home-made beef stock is not usually prepared for everyday meals, it will make all the difference when cooking something special.

Makes about 2.25 litres/4 pints

2.25 litres/4 pints water

2 ribs from cooked beef rib roast, fat trimmed

4 large onions, thickly sliced

4 medium carrots, thickly sliced

4 celery sticks, thickly sliced

1 parsnip, halved

2 bay leaves

8 black peppercorns

5 sage leaves

salt, to taste

Combine all the ingredients, except the salt, in a 5.5 litre/9½ pint slow cooker. Cover and cook on Low for 6–8 hours. Strain the stock through a double layer of muslin, discarding the solids. Season to taste with salt. Refrigerate until chilled. Remove the fat from the surface of the stock.

Fragrant Beef Stock

Dried mushrooms, red wine and herbs give a rich flavour to this stock. Brown the beef before adding it to the crock pot, if you like, for an even richer stock.

Makes about 3.25 litres/5¾ pints

2.75 litres/4¾ pints water
250 ml/8 fl oz dry red wine (optional)
900 g/2 lb short ribs of beef, fat trimmed
900 g/2 lb beef marrow bones
450 g/1 lb cubed chuck steak, fat trimmed
1 large onion, chopped
3 medium carrots, thickly sliced
3 celery sticks, thickly sliced
25 g/1 oz dried mushrooms
1 garlic clove, halved
10 black peppercorns
1 bay leaf
1 tsp dried basil
1 tsp thyme leaves
1 tbsp soy sauce
salt, to taste

Combine all the ingredients, except the salt, in a 5.5 litre/9½ pint slow cooker. Cover and cook on Low for 6–8 hours. Strain the stock through a double layer of muslin, discarding the solids. Season to taste with salt. Refrigerate until chilled. Remove the fat from the surface of the stock.

Veal Stock

Because veal bones can be difficult to find it's worth making this delicately flavoured stock when you can find the ingredients and then freezing it. Brown the veal for a richer flavour.

Makes about 2.25 litres/4 pints

2.25 litres/4 pints water
700 g/1½ lb veal cubes for stewing
1 onion, chopped
1 small carrot, chopped
1 small celery stick, chopped
1 veal knuckle or about 750 g/1¾ lb veal bones
2 bay leaves
6 black peppercorns
3 whole cloves
salt and freshly ground black pepper, to taste

Combine all the ingredients, except the salt and pepper, in a 5.5 litre/9½ pint slow cooker. Cover and cook on Low for 6–8 hours. Strain through a double layer of muslin, discarding the solids. Season to taste with salt and pepper. Refrigerate until chilled. Remove the fat from the surface of the stock.

Fish Stock

Ask your fishmonger or at the fish counter of your supermarket for bones to make this stock. If you use the fish heads, remove the gills first, as they can make the stock bitter.

Makes about 1.5 litres/2½ pints

1.5 litres/2½ pints water

900 g–1.5 kg/2–3 lb fish bones (from non-oily fish)

1 large onion, chopped

1 celery stick, chopped

2 bay leaves

7–8 black peppercorns

½ tsp sea salt

½ tsp white pepper

Combine all the ingredients in the slow cooker. Cook on Low for 4–6 hours. Strain through a double layer of muslin, discarding the solids.

Easy Fish Stock

Any mildly flavoured fish will make a delicious stock. Avoid strongly flavoured fish, such as salmon or tuna. Fish stock is best used on the day it is made, but it can also be frozen for up to 2 months.

Makes about 1 litre/1¾ pints

900 ml/1½ pints water

175 ml/6 fl oz dry white wine or water

700 g/1½ lb fresh or frozen fish steaks, cubed (2.5 cm/1 in)

1 onion, finely chopped

1 carrot, finely chopped

3 celery sticks with leaves, halved

3 sprigs of fresh parsley

3 lemon slices

8 black peppercorns

salt, to taste

Combine all the ingredients, except the salt, in the slow cooker. Cover and cook on Low for 4–6 hours. Strain the stock through a double layer of muslin, discarding the solids. Season to taste with salt.

Basic Vegetable Stock V

Perfect for vegetarian recipes, a good home-made stock gives a much rounder flavour than using a stock cube. As vegetables used in stocks are later discarded, they should be scrubbed but do not need to be peeled.

Makes about 2 litres/3½ pints

2 litres/3½ pints water
250 ml/8 fl oz dry white wine or water
1 large onion, thickly sliced
1 leek (white part only), thickly sliced
1 carrot, thickly sliced
1 celery stick, thickly sliced
450 g/1 lb mixed chopped vegetables (broccoli, French beans, cabbage, potatoes, tomatoes, courgettes or squash, peppers, mushrooms, etc.)
6–8 sprigs of fresh parsley
1 bay leaf
4 whole allspice
1 tbsp black peppercorns
2 tsp dried mixed herbs or 1 sachet of bouquet garni
salt, to taste

Combine all the ingredients, except the salt, in a 5.5 litre/9½ pint slow cooker. Cover and cook on Low for 6–8 hours. Strain the stock, discarding the solids. Season to taste with salt.

Roasted Vegetable Stock V

Roasting vegetables intensifies their flavours, adding richness to the stock. The beetroot adds a subtle sweetness to the stock, but only use it if you don't object to the pink colour it creates!

Makes about 2 litres/3½ pints

2 litres/3½ pints water

250 ml/8 fl oz dry white wine or water

1 medium onion, coarsely chopped

1 leek (white part only), coarsely chopped

1 carrot, coarsely chopped

1 courgette, coarsely chopped

1 turnip, coarsely chopped

1 beetroot, coarsely chopped

1 tomato, coarsely chopped

½ small butternut or acorn squash, cubed (5 cm/2 in)

1 garlic bulb, cut in half crosswise

175 g/6 oz kale, coarsely chopped

6 sprigs of fresh parsley

1 bay leaf

1–2 tsp dried mixed herbs or 1 sachet of bouquet garni

1 tsp black peppercorns

4 whole allspice

salt and freshly ground black pepper, to taste

Arrange the vegetables, except the kale, in a single layer on a greased, foil-lined Swiss roll tin. Bake at 220ºC/gas 7/fan oven 200ºC until tender and browned, 35–40 minutes.

Transfer the vegetables to a 5.5 litre/ 9½pint slow cooker and add the remaining ingredients, except the salt and pepper. Cover and cook on Low for 4–6 hours. Strain, discarding the solids. Season to taste with salt and pepper.

Mediterranean Stock V

A lovely stock, scented with orange and fennel. This is an unusual stock that will add richness to fresh soups and casseroles containing Mediterranean ingredients.

Makes about 2 litres/3½ pints

2 litres/3½ pints water

250 ml/8 fl oz dry white wine or water

juice of 1 orange

1 large onion, thickly sliced

1 leek (white part only), thickly sliced

1 carrot, thickly sliced

1 sweet potato, thickly sliced

1 courgette, thickly sliced

1 celery stick, thickly sliced

½ small fennel bulb, sliced

½ red pepper, sliced

2 medium tomatoes, quartered

1 medium garlic bulb, cut in half crosswise

225 g/8 oz coarsely chopped spinach or cos lettuce

6 sprigs of fresh parsley

1 strip of orange zest (7.5 cm/3 in x 2.5 cm/1 in)

1 bay leaf

1–2 tsp mixed herbs

1 tsp black peppercorns

4 whole allspice

salt, to taste

Combine all the ingredients, except the salt, in a 5.5 litre/9½ pint slow cooker. Cover and cook on Low for 4–6 hours. Strain, discarding the solids. Season to taste with salt.

Oriental Stock V

A light stock – fragrant with fresh coriander, ginger and five-spice powder – will bring Asian soups and entrées alive. Tamari is similar to soy sauce but with a smoother, richer taste.

Makes about 2 litres/3½ pints

2 litres/3½ pints water
350 g/12 oz pak choi or Chinese cabbage, shredded
65 g/2½ oz fresh coriander, coarsely chopped
1 large onion, sliced
1 carrot, sliced
1 small red pepper, sliced
5 cm/2 in fresh root ginger, sliced
3 large garlic cloves, crushed
3 dried shiitake mushrooms
4 tsp tamari
2 star anise
2 tsp Chinese five-spice powder
1½ tsp Szechuan peppercorns, toasted
salt and freshly ground black pepper, to taste

Combine all the ingredients, except the salt and pepper, in a 5.5 litre/9½ pint slow cooker. Cover and cook on Low for 4–6 hours. Strain, discarding the solids. Season to taste with salt and pepper.

Rich Mushroom Stock V

Dried shiitake mushrooms add richness and an unmistakeable depth of flavour to this stock.

Makes about 2 litres/3½ pints

1 litre/1¾ pints water

175 ml/6 fl oz dry white wine (optional)

1 large onion, sliced

1 leek (white part only), sliced

1 celery stick, sliced

350 g/12 oz button mushrooms

3 large garlic cloves, crushed

40–50 g/1½–2 oz dried shiitake mushrooms

6 sprigs of fresh parsley

¾ tsp dried sage

¾ tsp dried thyme

1½ tsp black peppercorns

salt, to taste

Combine all the ingredients, except the salt, in a 5.5 litre/9½ pint slow cooker. Cover and cook on Low for 6–8 hours. Strain, discarding the solids. Season to taste with salt and pepper.

Cream of Asparagus Soup V

A deliciously sophisticated dish for the asparagus season.

Serves 6

900 g/2 lb asparagus, cut into chunks

750 ml/1¼ pints vegetable stock

2 onions, chopped

3 garlic cloves, crushed

1 tsp dried marjoram

1 tsp grated lemon zest

a pinch of freshly grated nutmeg

120 ml/4 fl oz semi-skimmed milk

salt and white pepper, to taste

90 ml/6 tbsp soured cream

Reserve a few asparagus tips for garnish, then combine all the ingredients, except the milk, salt, white pepper and soured cream, in the slow cooker. Cover and cook on Low for 6–8 hours. Process the soup and milk in a food processor or blender until smooth. Season to taste with salt and white pepper. Serve warm or refrigerate and serve chilled. Top each bowl of soup with a dollop of soured cream.

Cream of Broccoli Soup V

Broccoli is a wonder food – high in antioxidants and packed with nutrients – and it has a lovely fresh taste too.

Serves 6

750 ml/1¼ pints vegetable stock
900 g/2 lb broccoli, cut into pieces (2.5 cm/1 in)
2 onions, chopped
3 garlic cloves, crushed
½ tsp dried thyme
a pinch of freshly grated nutmeg
120 ml/4 fl oz semi-skimmed milk
salt and white pepper, to taste
90 ml/6 tbsp soured cream
Crispy Croûtons (see below)

Combine all the ingredients, except the milk, salt, white pepper, soured cream and croûtons, in the slow cooker. Cover and cook on Low for 6–8 hours. Process the soup and milk in a food processor or blender until smooth. Season to taste with salt and white pepper. Serve warm or refrigerate and serve chilled. Top each bowl of soup with a dollop of soured cream and sprinkle with croûtons.

Crispy Croûtons V

The classic extra ideal for sprinkling on any soup.

Serves 6 as an accompaniment

3 slices firm or day-old French or Italian bread, cubed (1–2 cm/½–¾ in)

vegetable cooking spray

Spray the bread cubes with cooking spray. Arrange in a single layer on a baking tray. Bake at 190ºC/gas 5/fan oven 170ºC until browned, 8–10 minutes, stirring occasionally. Cool. Store in an airtight container for up to 2 weeks.

Broccoli and Dill Soup V

A great flavour combination – and a beautifully soft green colour.

Serves 6

750 ml/1¼ pints vegetable stock
900 g/2 lb broccoli, cut into pieces (2.5 cm/1 in)
2 onions, chopped
3 garlic cloves, crushed
30 ml/2 tbsp chopped fresh dill
120 ml/4 fl oz semi-skimmed milk
salt and white pepper, to taste
90 ml/6 tbsp soured cream

Combine the stock, broccoli, onions and garlic in the slow cooker. Cover and cook on Low for 6–8 hours. Add the fresh dill and milk and process the soup in a food processor or blender until smooth. Season to taste with salt and white pepper. Serve warm or refrigerate and serve chilled. Top each bowl of soup with a dollop of soured cream.

Broccoli and Kale Soup V

Kale is a slightly less common vegetable but you can buy it in most supermarkets.

Serves 6

750 ml/1¼ pints vegetable stock
900 g/2 lb broccoli, cut into pieces (2.5 cm/1 in)
2 onions, chopped
3 garlic cloves, crushed
½ tsp dried thyme
100 g/4 oz kale
salt and white pepper, to taste
90 ml/6 tbsp soured cream

Combine all the ingredients, except the kale, salt, white pepper and soured cream, in the slow cooker. Cover and cook on Low for 6–8 hours. Add the kale and cook for a further 15 minutes. Process the soup in a food processor or blender until smooth. Season to taste with salt and white pepper. Serve warm or refrigerate and serve chilled. Top each bowl of soup with a dollop of soured cream.

Broccoli and Cucumber Soup V

Most people don't think to cook with cucumber but you should give it a try.

Serves 6

750 ml/1¼ pints vegetable stock
900 g/2 lb broccoli, cut into pieces (2.5 cm/1 in)
1 cucumber, thickly sliced
2 onions, chopped
3 garlic cloves, crushed
25 g/1 oz fresh coriander, chopped
120 ml/4 fl oz semi-skimmed milk
salt and white pepper, to taste
90 ml/6 tbsp soured cream

Combine all the ingredients, except the milk, salt, white pepper and soured cream, in the slow cooker. Cover and cook on Low for 6–8 hours. Add the coriander and cook for a further 15 minutes. Process the soup and milk in a food processor or blender until smooth. Season to taste with salt and white pepper. Serve warm or refrigerate and serve chilled. Top each bowl of soup with a dollop of soured cream.

Creamy Broccoli and Potato Soup V

*Leeks add roundness to the flavour of this creamy soup. For a
colourful touch, garnish each bowl of soup with a lemon slice.*

Serves 6

750 ml/1¼ pints vegetable stock
2 broccoli heads, chopped
600 g/1 lb 6 oz potatoes, peeled and diced
4 medium leeks (white parts only), sliced
250 ml/8 fl oz milk
2 tbsp cornflour
salt and white pepper, to taste

Combine all the ingredients, except the milk, cornflour, salt and
pepper, in the slow cooker and cook on Low for 6–8 hours. Stir in
the combined milk and cornflour, stirring until thickened, 2–3
minutes. Process the soup in a food processor or blender until
smooth. Season to taste with salt and white pepper.

Herbed Broccoli and Cauliflower Bisque

The unmistakeable taste of basil goes surprisingly well with broccoli and cauliflower.

Serves 6

750 ml/1¼ pints vegetable stock

2 heads of broccoli, coarsely chopped

½ small head of cauliflower, coarsely chopped

250 g/9 oz potatoes, peeled and coarsely chopped

8 spring onions, thinly sliced

1 tbsp dried basil

250 ml/8 fl oz milk

salt and freshly ground black pepper, to taste

Combine all the ingredients, except the milk, salt and pepper, in the slow cooker. Cover and cook on High for 4–5 hours. Process the soup and milk in a food processor or blender until smooth. Season to taste with salt and pepper.

Hot-and-sour Cabbage Soup V

Oriental chilli oil adds to the authentic flavour of this soup, a slow-cooker version of the classic Chinese dish.

Serves 4

1.2 litres/3 pints vegetable stock
75 g/3 oz green cabbage, shredded
1 small carrot, chopped
¼ red pepper, finely chopped
2 spring onions, thinly sliced
1 small garlic clove, crushed
1 tsp finely grated fresh root ginger
1½ tbsp soy sauce
2 tsp cider vinegar
a dash of oriental hot chilli oil
1 tbsp cornflour
½ tbsp light brown sugar

Combine the stock, vegetables, garlic and ginger in the slow cooker. Cover and cook on Low for 6–8 hours. Stir in the combined remaining ingredients during the last 2–3 minutes.

Dilled Carrot Soup V

Carrot soup is always a favourite, whether hot or chilled. Here carrots are teamed with dill for a fresh, clean flavour.

Serves 6

750 ml/1¼ pints vegetable stock
400 g/14 oz can chopped tomatoes
450 g/1 lb carrots, thickly sliced
3 onions, chopped
1 medium floury potato, peeled and cubed
2 garlic cloves, crushed
1–1½ tsp dried dill
2–3 tbsp lemon juice
salt and white pepper, to taste
90 ml/6 tbsp plain yoghurt

Combine all the ingredients, except the lemon juice, salt, white pepper and yoghurt, in the slow cooker. Cover and cook on Low 6–8 hours. Process the soup in a food processor or blender until smooth. Season to taste with lemon juice, salt and white pepper. Serve the soup warm or refrigerate and serve chilled. Garnish each bowl of soup with a dollop of yoghurt.

Cream of Cauliflower Soup with Cheese V

The family favourite, cauliflower cheese, but in a bowl! This puréed soup has a velvety texture and is perfect for lunch or a first course.

Serves 6

900 ml/1½ pints vegetable stock
350 g/12 oz cauliflower, cut into florets
1 large floury potato, peeled and cubed
1 onion, chopped
2 garlic cloves, crushed
120 ml/4 fl oz semi-skimmed milk
1 tbsp cornflour
75 g/3 oz Cheddar cheese, grated
salt and white pepper, to taste
ground mace or freshly grated nutmeg, to garnish

Combine the stock, cauliflower, potato, onion and garlic in the slow cooker. Cover and cook on Low for 6–8 hours. Remove about half the vegetables from the soup with a slotted spoon and reserve. Purée the remaining soup in a food processor or blender until smooth. Return to the slow cooker. Add the reserved vegetables. Cover and cook on High for 10 minutes. Stir in the combined milk and cornflour, stirring for 2–3 minutes. Add the cheese, stirring until melted. Season to taste with salt and white pepper. Sprinkle each bowl of soup with mace or nutmeg.

Chilled Cauliflower Soup V

The addition of fragrant, fresh-flavoured dill makes this a lovely soup for a summer lunch.

Serves 6

900 ml/1½ pints vegetable stock
350 g/12 oz cauliflower, cut into florets
1 large floury potato, peeled and cubed
1 onion, chopped
2 garlic cloves, crushed
120 ml/4 fl oz semi-skimmed milk
1 tbsp dried dill
salt and white pepper, to taste
chopped fresh dill or parsley, to garnish

Combine the stock, cauliflower, potato, onion and garlic in the slow cooker. Cover and cook on Low for 6–8 hours. Purée the soup with the milk and dried dill in a food processor or blender until smooth. Season to taste with salt and white pepper. Serve chilled, garnished with fresh dill or parsley.

Courgette Soup V

A perfect soup for that summer glut of courgettes. It can also be made with marrow or patty pan squash.

Serves 6

750 ml/1¼ pints vegetable stock
4 medium courgettes, chopped
275 g/10 oz floury potato, peeled and cubed
75 g/3 oz chopped shallots
3 spring onions, chopped
2 garlic cloves, crushed
1½ tsp dried tarragon
50 g/2 oz chopped kale or spinach
120 ml/4 fl oz semi-skimmed milk
1 tbsp cornflour
salt and white pepper, to taste
cayenne pepper, to garnish
Garlic Croûtons (see below)

Combine the stock, courgettes, potato, shallots, onions, garlic and tarragon in the slow cooker. Cover and cook on High for 4–5 hours, adding the kale and combined milk and cornflour during the last 15 minutes. Process the soup in a food processor or blender until smooth. Season to taste with salt and white pepper. Serve warm or chilled. Sprinkle each bowl of soup with cayenne pepper and top with Garlic Croûtons.

Garlic Croûtons V

Delicious and crunchy with a hint of garlic – or more if you like!

Serves 6 as an accompaniment

3 slices firm or day-old French bread, cubed (1 cm/½ in)
vegetable cooking spray
1 tsp garlic powder

Spray the bread cubes with cooking spray. Sprinkle with garlic powder and toss. Arrange in single layer on a baking tray. Bake at 190ºC/gas 5/fan oven 170ºC until browned, 8–10 minutes, stirring occasionally.

Courgette Soup with Garlic and Curry V

Lots of garlic, and a hint of curry and marjoram enliven courgettes in this wonderful summer soup.

Serves 8

1 litre/1¾ pints vegetable stock

500 g/18 oz courgettes, sliced

4 onions, chopped

4 garlic cloves, crushed

2 tbsp tarragon vinegar

2 tsp curry powder

1 tsp dried marjoram

¼ tsp celery seeds

120 ml/4 fl oz plain yoghurt

salt and cayenne pepper, to taste

paprika, to garnish

Combine all the ingredients, except the yoghurt, salt, cayenne pepper and paprika, in the slow cooker. Cover and cook on Low for 6–8 hours. Process the soup and yoghurt in a food processor or blender until smooth. Season to taste with salt and cayenne pepper. Serve warm or refrigerate and serve chilled. Sprinkle each bowl of soup with paprika.

Fennel Bisque with Walnuts

The delicate aniseed flavour of fennel makes a delicious soup.

Serves 6

900 ml/1½ pints vegetable stock

350 g/12 oz fennel bulbs, sliced

1 large floury potato, peeled and cubed

1 large leek, sliced

2 garlic cloves, crushed

120 ml/4 fl oz semi-skimmed milk

salt and white pepper, to taste

50 g/2 oz blue cheese, crumbled

50 g/2 oz walnuts, toasted and chopped

Combine the stock, fennel, potato, leek and garlic in the slow cooker. Cover and cook on Low for 6–8 hours. Purée the soup and milk in a food processor or blender until smooth. Return to the slow cooker. Season to taste with salt and white pepper. Sprinkle each bowl of soup with blue cheese and walnuts to serve.

Garlic Soup with Toasted Bread V

Long, slow cooking mellows the pungency of garlic, making it gorgeously rich. A beaten egg can be stirred into the soup before serving.

Serves 4

1 litre/1¾ pints vegetable stock
6–8 garlic cloves, finely chopped
½ tsp ground cumin
½ tsp dried oregano
salt and cayenne pepper, to taste
4 slices French or sourdough bread
vegetable cooking spray
chopped fresh coriander, to garnish

Combine the stock, garlic, cumin and oregano in the slow cooker. Cover and cook on High for 4 hours. Season to taste with salt and cayenne pepper.

Spray both sides of the bread slices generously with cooking spray. Cook in a frying pan over medium heat until golden, about 2 minutes on each side. Place a slice of bread in each soup bowl. Ladle the soup over and sprinkle with coriander.

Fragrant Mushroom Soup

An important element of this soup's success is the Fragrant Beef Stock, which really makes it something special.

Serves 4

550 g/1¼ lb mushrooms

750 ml/1¼ pints Fragrant Beef Stock or beef stock

1 tbsp light soy sauce

2 tbsp cornflour

50 ml/2 fl oz water

2 tbsp dry sherry (optional)

½ tsp lemon juice

salt and freshly ground black pepper, to taste

Slice 100 g/4 oz of the mushrooms and reserve. Coarsely chop the remaining mushrooms and stalks. Combine the chopped mushrooms, stock and soy sauce in the slow cooker. Cover and cook on Low for 4–6 hours. Process the soup in a food processor or blender until smooth. Return to the slow cooker. Add the sliced mushrooms. Cover and cook on High for 30 minutes. Stir in the combined cornflour and water, stirring for 2–3 minutes. Stir in the sherry and lemon juice. Season to taste with salt and pepper.

Lemon Mushroom Soup

Fresh and dried mushrooms combine in this richly flavoured, lemon-accented soup.

Serves 6

375 ml/13 fl oz hot water

25 g/1 oz dried porcini or other dried mushrooms

750 ml/1¼ pints Rich Chicken Stock or chicken or vegetable stock

50 ml/2 fl oz dry white wine (optional)

225 g/8 oz brown cap mushrooms, quartered

1 onion, thinly sliced

4 large garlic cloves, crushed

1 tsp dried rosemary leaves

flesh of ½ lemon, chopped

15 g/½ oz parsley, chopped

50 ml/2 fl oz water

2 tbsp cornflour

salt and freshly ground black pepper, to taste

Bruschetta (see below)

Pour the hot water over the porcini mushrooms in a bowl. Leave to stand until softened, about 20 minutes. Remove the mushrooms with a slotted spoon. Strain the liquid through a double layer of muslin and reserve. Inspect the mushrooms carefully, rinsing if necessary, to remove any grit. Chop coarsely.

Combine the porcini mushrooms and reserved liquid with the remaining ingredients, except the lemon, parsley, water, cornflour, salt, pepper and Bruschetta, in the slow cooker. Cover and cook on Low for 6–8 hours, adding the lemon and parsley during the last 5 minutes. Stir in the combined water and cornflour for 2–3 minutes. Season to taste with salt and pepper. Place a Bruschetta in each soup bowl and ladle the soup over.

Bruschetta V

Delicious with so many recipes, this is particularly happy with Mediterranean-style flavours.

Makes 6

6 slices French bread (2 cm/¾ in)
olive oil cooking spray
1 garlic clove, halved

Spray both sides of the bread lightly with cooking spray. Grill on a baking sheet 3 cm/1¼ in from the heat source, until browned, 2–3 minutes on each side. Rub the top sides of the bread with the cut sides of the garlic.

White Onion Soup V

The mild sweetness of white onions makes this soup different, but try it with other onion varieties too. For a richer flavour, brown the onions in a frying pan before adding to the slow cooker.

Serves 8

1.5 litres/2½ pints vegetable stock
6 large white onions, thinly sliced
2 garlic cloves, crushed
1 tsp sugar
1½ tsp dried sage
2 bay leaves
2–3 tbsp cornflour
50 ml/2 fl oz water
salt and white pepper, to taste
snipped chives or sliced spring onions, to garnish

Combine all the ingredients, except the cornflour, water, salt and white pepper in a 5.5 litre/9½ pint slow cooker. Cover and cook on High for 5–6 hours. Discard the bay leaves. Stir in the combined cornflour and water, stirring for 2–3 minutes. Process the soup in a food processor or blender until smooth. Season to taste with salt and white pepper. Serve warm or chilled. Sprinkle each bowl of soup with chives or spring onion.

Three-onion Soup with Mushrooms V

For a soup with a richer flavour, sprinkle the onions, leeks and shallots with 1 tsp sugar and cook in 1 tbsp butter in a large frying pan over medium-low heat until the onions are golden, about 15 minutes.

Serves 6

1.5 litres/2½ pints vegetable stock
6 onions, thinly sliced
2 small leeks, thinly sliced
150 g/5 oz shallots or spring onions, chopped
175 g/6 oz mushrooms, sliced
1 tsp sugar
salt and freshly ground black pepper, to taste

Combine all the ingredients, except the salt and pepper, in the slow cooker. Cover and cook on Low for 6–8 hours. Season to taste with salt and pepper.

Red Onion and Apple Soup with Curry

Slow cooking brings out the sweetness of red onions, lending a well-rounded flavour to this autumn soup.

Serves 6

1.5 litres/2½ pints Rich Chicken Stock or chicken or vegetable stock

550 g/1¼ lb red onions, thinly sliced

4 tart cooking apples, peeled and coarsely grated

1 carrot, cubed (1 cm/½ in)

1 large bay leaf

1 tsp curry powder

1 tsp chilli powder

¼ tsp dried thyme

¼ tsp ground allspice

salt and freshly ground black pepper, to taste

mango chutney, to garnish

Combine all the ingredients, except the salt and pepper, in the slow cooker. Cover and cook on High for 4–5 hours. Discard the bay leaf. Season to taste with salt and pepper. Serve with chutney to stir into the soup.

Onion and Leek Soup with Pasta V

All the flavour and health-giving properties of these vegetables from the allium family are found in a bowl of this soup. You're spoilt for choice when it comes to suitable pasta shapes to use. Soup pasta, farfalle or conchiglie are all good.

Serves 6

1.75 litres/3 pints vegetable stock

8 onions, sliced

2 medium leeks (white parts only), sliced

6 garlic cloves, crushed

1 tsp sugar

100 g/4 oz pasta, cooked

salt and white pepper, to taste

6 tsp freshly grated Parmesan cheese

Combine all the ingredients, except the pasta, salt, white pepper and Parmesan cheese, in the slow cooker. Cover and cook on High for 4–5 hours, adding the pasta during the last 20 minutes. Season to taste with salt and white pepper. Sprinkle each bowl of soup with 1 tsp Parmesan cheese.

Canadian Pea Soup

A delicious version of this well-known classic.

Serves 4

1.2 litres/2 pints water

225 g/8 oz dried yellow split peas

50 g /2 oz diced lean salt pork

1 small onion, quartered

1 leek (white part only), sliced

1 carrot, sliced

1 small parsnip, cubed

1 large tomato, chopped

1 garlic cloves, crushed

2 whole cloves

1 tsp dried thyme

1 bay leaf

salt and freshly ground black pepper, to taste

Combine all the ingredients, except the salt and pepper, in the slow cooker. Cover and cook on Low for 6–8 hours. Discard the bay leaf. Season to taste with salt and pepper.

Hot Chilli Vichyssoise V

Potato soup will never be boring if served Tex-Mex style. This version, prepared with chillies, certainly packs a punch!

Serves 6

1 litre/1¾ pints vegetable stock

450 g/1 lb new red potatoes, unpeeled, halved

1 medium leek (white part only), sliced

1 poblano chilli, very finely chopped

1 jalapeño or other medium-hot chilli, very finely chopped

6 garlic cloves, peeled

1½ tsp ground cumin

½ tsp chilli powder

½ tsp dried oregano

175 ml/6 fl oz semi-skimmed milk

1 tbsp cornflour

10 g/¼ oz chopped fresh coriander

salt, to taste

Combine all the ingredients, except the milk, cornflour, coriander and salt, in a 5.5 litre/9½ pint slow cooker. Cover and cook on High for 4–5 hours. Stir in the combined milk and cornflour, stirring for 2–3 minutes. Process the soup in a food processor or blender until smooth. Stir in the coriander. Season with salt. Serve warm or chilled.

Ginger Pumpkin Soup V

Bright pumpkin with a hint of ginger – lovely! Yellow winter squash, such as butternut or onion, can be substituted for the pumpkin.

Serves 6

750 ml/1¼ pints vegetable stock

1 small pumpkin (about 900 g/2 lb), peeled, seeded and cubed

2 onions, chopped

1 tbsp chopped fresh root ginger

1 tsp crushed garlic

120 ml/4 fl oz dry white wine, or vegetable stock

½ tsp ground cloves

salt and freshly ground black pepper, to taste

Combine all the ingredients, except the salt and pepper, in the slow cooker. Cover and cook on High for 4–5 hours. Process the soup in a food processor or blender until smooth. Season to taste with salt and pepper.

Spinach and Pasta Soup with Basil V

Chickpeas and spinach are comfortable Mediterranean partners. Here they are served in a soup flavoured with basil. Serve with garlic bread or focaccia.

Serves 4

1.5 litres/2½ pints vegetable stock
1 small onion, finely chopped
1 crushed garlic clove
1–1½ tsp dried basil leaves
75 g/3 oz chopped plum tomatoes, fresh or canned
150 g/5 oz drained canned chickpeas, rinsed
275 g/10 oz frozen chopped spinach, thawed
75 g/3 oz vermicelli, broken and cooked
salt and freshly ground black pepper, to taste
2 tbsp freshly grated Parmesan cheese, to garnish

Combine all the ingredients, except the spinach, pasta, salt and pepper, in the slow cooker. Cover and cook on High for 4–6 hours, adding the spinach and pasta during the last 30 minutes. Season to taste with salt and pepper. Sprinkle each bowl of soup with Parmesan cheese.

Spinach and Pasta Soup with Ham and Beans

This makes a substantial first-course soup, so team with a light main course.

Serves 4

1.5 litres/2½ pints vegetable or chicken stock

225–350 g/8–12 oz boneless pork loin, cubed

1 small onion, finely chopped

1 crushed garlic clove

1–1½ tsp dried basil leaves

75 g/3 oz chopped plum tomatoes, fresh or canned

150 g/5 oz drained canned haricot or cannellini beans, rinsed

275 g/10 oz frozen chopped spinach, thawed

75 g/3 oz vermicelli, broken and cooked

salt and freshly ground black pepper, to taste

2 tbsp freshly grated Parmesan cheese, to garnish

Combine all the ingredients, except the spinach, pasta, salt and pepper, in the slow cooker. Cover and cook on High for 4–6 hours, adding the spinach and pasta during the last 30 minutes. Season to taste with salt and pepper. Sprinkle each bowl of soup with Parmesan cheese.

Acorn Squash Soup V

Sweet spices complement this autumn soup, making it especially warming. It will also work well with any winter squash or pumpkin.

Serves 6

450 ml/¾ pint vegetable stock

2 medium acorn squash, peeled and cubed

1 onion, chopped

½ tsp ground cinnamon

¼ tsp ground coriander

¼ tsp cumin

120 ml/4 fl oz semi-skimmed milk

1 tbsp cider vinegar

salt and freshly ground black pepper, to taste

Combine all the ingredients, except the milk, vinegar, salt and pepper, in the slow cooker. Cover and cook on Low for 6–8 hours. Process the soup, milk and vinegar in a food processor or blender until smooth. Season to taste with salt and pepper.

Apple Squash Soup V

This soup is the perfect autumn offering, combining the newly ripened squashes with the bright flavour of cider, and enlivened with spices.

Serves 8

750 ml/1¼ pints vegetable stock
350 ml/12 fl oz cider
1 large butternut squash (about 1.25 kg/2½ lb), peeled, seeded and cubed
2 tart cooking apples, peeled, cored and chopped
3 onions, chopped
2 tsp ground cinnamon
¼ tsp ground ginger,
¼ tsp ground cloves
a pinch of freshly grated nutmeg
salt and freshly ground black pepper, to taste
Spiced Soured Cream (see below)

Combine all the ingredients, except the salt, pepper and Spiced Soured Cream, in the slow cooker. Cover and cook on High for 4–5 hours. Process the soup in a food processor or blender until smooth. Season to taste with salt and pepper. Serve with Spiced Soured Cream.

Spiced Soured Cream V

This gently spicy cream goes particularly well with oriental soups.

Serves 8 as an accompaniment

120 ml/4 fl oz soured cream

1 tsp sugar

½ tsp ground cinnamon

a pinch of ground ginger

1–2 tsp lemon juice

Combine all the ingredients.

Squash and Fennel Bisque V

A delicious soup – you can thin with additional stock if necessary.

Serves 6

750 ml/1¼ pints vegetable stock
1 fennel bulb, sliced
1 celery stick, sliced
275 g/10 oz floury potato, peeled and cubed
75 g/3 oz chopped shallots
3 spring onions, chopped
2 garlic cloves, crushed
50 g/2 oz chopped spinach
120 ml/4 fl oz semi-skimmed milk
1 tbsp cornflour
salt and white pepper, to taste
cayenne pepper, to garnish
Garlic Croûtons

Combine the stock, fennel, celery, potato, shallots, onions and garlic in the slow cooker. Cover and cook on High for 4–5 hours, adding the kale and blended milk and flour during the last 15 minutes. Process the soup in a food processor or blender until smooth. Season to taste with salt and white pepper. Serve warm or chilled. Sprinkle each bowl of soup with cayenne pepper and top with Garlic Croûtons.

Cream of Tomato Soup

A soup similar to the favourite brand-name canned tomato soup we all remember eating as kids. Canned tomatoes are necessary for the flavour, so don't substitute fresh.

Serves 4

450 ml/¾ pint full-fat milk

400 g/14 oz can chopped tomatoes

1–2 tsp beef bouillon granules, or a beef stock cube

3 tbsp cornflour

a pinch of bicarbonate of soda

2 tsp sugar

25 g/1 oz butter or margarine

salt and freshly ground black pepper, to taste

Combine 250 ml/8 fl oz milk, the tomatoes and bouillon granules in the slow cooker. Cover and cook on Low for 3–4 hours. Process in a food processor or blender until smooth, then return to the slow cooker. Cover and cook on High for 10 minutes. Stir in the combined remaining milk and the cornflour, stirring for 2–3 minutes. Stir in the bicarbonate of soda, sugar and butter or margarine. Season to taste with salt and pepper.

Winter Gazpacho

This hot version of gazpacho brings vegetable-garden flavours and a bright assortment of garnishes to the winter dinner table.

Serves 6

1 litre/1¾ pints tomato juice

1 carrot, chopped

1 celery stick, chopped

½ green pepper, chopped

2 tsp Worcestershire sauce

1 tsp beef bouillon granules, or a beef stock cube

¼ tsp dried tarragon

75 g/3 oz spinach

salt and cayenne pepper, to taste

1 small onion, chopped

1 hard-boiled egg

1 small avocado, cubed

Garlic Croûtons

Combine the tomato juice, carrot, celery, pepper, Worcestershire sauce, bouillon granules and tarragon in the slow cooker. Cover and cook on High for 4–5 hours adding the spinach during the last 15 minutes. Process the soup in a food processor or blender until smooth. Season to taste with salt and cayenne pepper. Serve in shallow bowls. Sprinkle with chopped onion, egg, avocado and Garlic Croûtons.

Two-tomato Soup V

The concentrated flavour of sun-dried tomatoes enhances the taste of garden-ripe tomato soup.

Serves 6

1 litre/1¾ pints vegetable stock

700 g/1½ lb chopped ripe or canned tomatoes

2 onions, chopped

1 celery stick, chopped

1 carrot, chopped

2 tsp crushed garlic cloves

1 large floury potato, peeled and cubed

25 g/1 oz sun-dried tomatoes (not in oil), at room temperature

½ tsp dried basil leaves

120 ml/4 fl oz semi-skimmed milk

2–3 tsp sugar

salt and freshly ground black pepper, to taste

Combine all the ingredients, except the milk, sugar, salt and pepper, in the slow cooker. Cover and cook on High for 4–5 hours. Process the soup and milk in a food processor or blender until smooth. Season to taste with sugar, salt and pepper.

Baked Two-tomato Soup V

This makes a very impressive starter for a dinner party.

Serves 6

1 quantity Two-tomato Soup (see above)
375 g/13 oz ready-rolled puff pastry
1 egg, beaten
2 tbsp freshly grated Parmesan cheese

Make the soup as above and ladle into ovenproof bowls. Cut the pastry into 6 rounds just a little larger than the size of the tops of the bowls. Moisten the edges of the pastry with egg and place on top of the bowls, pressing gently over the rims. Brush with egg and sprinkle each with 1–2 tsp freshly grated Parmesan cheese. Bake at 190ºC/gas 5/fan oven 170ºC until the pastry is puffed and golden, about 20 minutes.

Smoky Tomato Bisque

Smoked pork hocks and a wide range of vegetables, herbs and spices give a rich and full flavour to this tomato soup.

Serves 8

600 ml/1 pint beef stock

2 x 400 g/14 oz cans chopped tomatoes

175 g/6 oz tomato purée

2 small smoked pork hocks

1 large onion, chopped

1 potato, peeled and cubed

1 carrot, sliced

1 small red pepper

2 celery sticks, sliced

2 garlic cloves, crushed

1 tsp dried thyme

½ tsp ground allspice

½ tsp curry powder

375 ml/13 fl oz full-fat milk

2 tbsp cornflour

1 tsp sugar

salt and freshly ground black pepper, to taste

Combine all the ingredients, except the milk, cornflour, sugar, salt and pepper, in the slow cooker. Cover and cook on High for 4–5 hours. Discard the pork hocks. Process the soup and 250 ml/8 fl oz milk in a food processor or blender until smooth. Return to the slow cooker. Cover and cook on High for 10 minutes. Stir in the combined remaining milk, the cornflour and sugar, stirring for 2–3 minutes. Season to taste with salt and pepper.

Zesty Tomato and Vegetable Soup

Italian tomatoes make this flavourful vegetable soup with a hint of chilli especially good.

Serves 6

450 ml/¾ pint beef stock

2 x 400 g/14 oz cans Italian plum tomatoes

50 ml/2 fl oz dry white wine

1 tsp lemon juice

1 onion, chopped

1 large celery stick, chopped

1 carrot, chopped

1 red pepper, chopped

¾ tsp celery salt

a pinch of crushed chilli flakes

salt and freshly ground black pepper, to taste

Combine all the ingredients, except the salt and pepper, in the slow cooker. Cover and cook on High for 4–5 hours. Process the soup in a food processor or blender until smooth. Season to taste with salt and pepper. Serve warm or refrigerate and serve chilled.

Cream of Turnip Soup V

A much underrated vegetable, this recipe really brings out the flavour.

Serves 6

900 ml/1½ pints vegetable stock
350 g/12 oz turnips, chopped
1 large floury potato, peeled and cubed
1 onion, chopped
2 garlic cloves, crushed
120 ml/4 fl oz semi-skimmed milk
1 tbsp cornflour
75 g/3 oz Swiss cheese, grated
½ tsp dried thyme
salt and white pepper, to taste
ground mace or freshly grated nutmeg, to garnish

Combine the stock, turnips, potato, onion and garlic in the slow cooker. Cover and cook on Low for 6–8 hours. Purée the soup, milk, cornflour, cheese and thyme in a food processor or blender until smooth. Season to taste with salt and white pepper. Sprinkle each bowl of soup with mace or nutmeg.

Garden Soup V

A light, colourful soup, which showcases an appealing blend of vegetables.

Serves 6

1 litre/1¾ pints vegetable stock

2 onions, chopped

150 g/5 oz drained, canned cannellini beans, rinsed

½ red pepper, diced

1 celery stick, diced

1 carrot, diced

2 garlic cloves, crushed

1 bay leaf

1½ tsp dried Italian herb seasoning

65 g/2½ oz diced yellow summer squash, such as patty pan

65 g/2½ oz courgettes

2 medium tomatoes, diced

salt and freshly ground black pepper, to taste

Combine all the ingredients, except the squash, courgettes, tomatoes, salt and pepper, in the slow cooker. Cover and cook on Low for 6–8 hours, adding the squash, courgettes and tomatoes during the last 30 minutes. Discard the bay leaf. Season to taste with salt and pepper.

Many-vegetable Soup V

Asparagus, mushrooms and broccoli team with traditional soup vegetables to make an unusual and delightful combination. You can use any vegetables you like, so It's an ideal soup to make when you need to use up leftovers in the fridge.

Serves 4

450 ml/¾ pint vegetable stock
½ tsp dried tarragon
1 carrot, coarsely chopped
1 celery stick, coarsely chopped
1 onion, coarsely chopped
50 g/2 oz mushrooms, coarsely chopped
100 g/4 oz small broccoli florets, coarsely chopped
175 g/6 oz asparagus, sliced (2.5 cm/1 in)
250 ml/8 fl oz plain yoghurt
2 tbsp cornflour
salt and freshly ground black pepper, to taste

Combine the stock, tarragon and vegetables, except the asparagus, in the slow cooker. Cover and cook on Low for 6–8 hours, adding the asparagus during the last 20 minutes. Stir in the combined yoghurt and cornflour, stirring for 2–3 minutes. Season to taste with salt and pepper.

Stracciatelle with Mini-meatballs

Turkey Meatballs are a real treat when served mini-size with a tasty soup. When you stir the egg whites into the hot soup they look like threads or, in Italian, stracciatelle – 'torn rags'.

Serves 4

1 litre/1¾ pints chicken stock

100 g/4 oz spinach, sliced

Turkey Meatballs (see below)

1 celery stick, chopped

1 onion, chopped

1 carrot, sliced

50 g/2 oz pastina or other small soup pasta

1 egg white, lightly beaten

salt and freshly ground black pepper, to taste

shaved Parmesan cheese, to garnish

Combine all the ingredients, except the pasta, egg white, salt and pepper, in the slow cooker. Cover and cook on Low for 6–8 hours, adding the pasta during the last 30 minutes. Slowly stir the egg white into the soup. Season to taste with salt and pepper. Garnish each bowl of soup with Parmesan cheese.

Turkey Meatballs

These tasty little meatballs can be added to any number of soups but particularly suit fairly substantial ones.

Makes 24 meatballs

225 g/8 oz lean minced turkey

½ small onion, very finely chopped

2 tbsp seasoned dry breadcrumbs

1 tbsp freshly grated Parmesan cheese

2 tbsp tomato purée

Combine all the ingredients in a bowl. Shape the mixture into 24 small meatballs and add to the soup before cooking.

Vegetable and Barley Soup

Pearl barley is a traditional addition to soups, and here it enhances a tomato-based soup of beans, potatoes and cabbage. Any vegetables you like can be substituted for those listed.

Serves 8

2.25 litres/4 pints beef stock

400 g/14 oz ready-made tomato sauce

350 g/12 oz potatoes, peeled and cubed

275 g/10 oz French beans, cut into short lengths

225 g/8 oz cabbage, thinly sliced

25 g/1 oz finely chopped parsley

1 tbsp dried Italian herb seasoning

1–2 tsp chilli powder

65 g/2½ oz pearl barley

salt and freshly ground black pepper, to taste

Combine all the ingredients, except the barley, salt and pepper, in a 5.5 litre/9½ pint slow cooker. Cover and cook on High for 2 hours. Add the barley and cook for 2 hours. Season to taste with salt and pepper.

Bean and Barley Soup with Kale

This nutritious soup with a gentle spike of chilli is a great start to any meal.

Serves 8

1.75 litres/3 pints Fragrant Beef Stock or beef stock

2 x 400 g/14 oz cans cannellini beans, rinsed and drained

3 onions, chopped

1 large carrot, chopped

225 g/8 oz mushrooms, sliced

1 tsp crushed garlic

¼ tsp crushed chilli flakes, to taste

2 tsp dried thyme

90 g/3½ oz pearl barley

225 g/8 oz sliced kale

1 tbsp lemon juice

salt and freshly ground black pepper, to taste

Combine all the ingredients, except the barley, kale, lemon juice, salt and pepper, in a 5.5 litre/9½ pint slow cooker. Cover and cook on High for 2–3 hours. Add the barley and cook for 2 hours, adding the kale during the last 30 minutes. Stir in the lemon juice. Season to taste with salt and pepper.

Haricot Bean and Spinach Soup

*A delicious, hearty soup with the meaty taste of smoked pork and a
wholesome flavour created by lots of vegetables.*

Serves 6

2.25 litres/4 pints chicken stock

1 smoked pork hock (optional)

275g/10 oz dried haricot beans, rinsed

1 large chopped onion

2 garlic cloves, crushed

2 large carrots, sliced

2 celery sticks, sliced

2 bay leaves

¾ tsp dried marjoram

¾ tsp dried thyme

¾ tsp dried basil

50 g/2 oz pearl barley

400 g/14 oz can tomatoes

275 g/10 oz frozen chopped spinach, thawed

salt and cayenne pepper, to taste

Combine all the ingredients, except the barley, tomatoes, spinach,
salt and cayenne pepper, in a 5.5 litre/9½ pint slow cooker. Cover
and cook on Low until the beans are tender, 6–8 hours. Add the
barley and cook for 2 hours, adding the tomatoes and spinach

during the last 30 minutes. Discard the pork hock and bay leaves. Season to taste with salt and cayenne pepper.

Lentil Soup

This satisfying soup is good on a cold day – and it's quick to prepare. Lentils have a good savoury flavour and work exceptionally well cooked this way.

Serves 6

2.25 litres/4 pints water

1 large smoked pork hock

450 g/1 lb dried brown lentils

2 onions, finely chopped

1 celery stick, finely chopped

1 carrot, finely chopped

2 tsp sugar,

2 tsp beef bouillon granules, or a beef stock cube

¼ tsp dry mustard powder

½ tsp dried thyme

salt and cayenne pepper, to taste

Combine all the ingredients, except the salt and cayenne pepper, in a 5.5 litre/9½ pint slow cooker. Cover and cook on Low for 6–8 hours. Discard the pork hock. Season to taste with salt and cayenne pepper.

Lentil Soup with Orzo

The rice-shaped pasta called orzo makes a simple soup exciting

Serves 6

450 ml/¾ pint beef stock

2 x 400 g/14 oz cans plum tomatoes

250 ml/8 fl oz water

225 g/8 oz dried lentils

4 onions, minced or very finely chopped

1 large carrot, chopped

1 large celery stick, chopped

3 large garlic cloves, crushed

1 tsp dried oregano leaves

¼ tsp crushed chilli flakes

100 g/4 oz orzo or other small soup pasta

175 g/6 oz spinach, sliced

salt and freshly ground black pepper, to taste

Combine all the ingredients, except the orzo, spinach, salt and pepper, in a 5.5 litre/9½ pint slow cooker. Cover and cook on High for 4–5 hours, adding the orzo and spinach during the last 30 minutes. Season to taste with salt and pepper.

Sausage and Lentil Soup

A thick and hearty soup accented with the robust taste of sausage. Use any sausages you like. You could even try some game sausages for a more pronounced flavour.

Serves 4

175 g/6 oz good-quality pork or beef sausage, casings removed
1.5 litres/2½ pints beef stock
200 g/7 oz chopped tomatoes
225 g/8 oz red lentils
2 onions, chopped
1 medium carrot, chopped
½ tsp dried thyme
1 small bay leaf
1 tsp lemon juice
salt and freshly ground black pepper, to taste

Cook the sausage in a frying pan over medium heat, crumbling with a fork, until browned, about 8 minutes. Combine the sausage and the remaining ingredients, except the lemon juice, salt and pepper, in a 5.5 litre/9½ pint slow cooker. Cover and cook on Low for 6–8 hours. Discard the bay leaf. Season to taste with lemon juice, salt and pepper.

Lentil Soup with Fennel

Use vegetable stock instead of beef if you want to make a vegetarian version of this tasty, lentil-based soup.

Serves 4

1 small fennel bulb, sliced

1.5 litres/2 ½ pints beef stock

200 g/7 oz chopped tomatoes

225 g/8 oz red lentils

2 onions, chopped

1 medium carrot, chopped

½ tsp crushed fennel seeds

1 small bay leaf

1 tsp lemon juice

salt and freshly ground black pepper, to taste

Reserve a few fennel fronds and chop them coarsely. Combine the ingredients, except the lemon juice, salt and pepper, in the slow cooker. Cover and cook on Low for 6–8 hours. Discard the bay leaf. Season to taste with lemon juice, salt and pepper. Garnish with the reserved fennel tops.

Dutch Split Pea Soup

A rich and delicious treat.

Serves 4

1.2 litres/2 pints water

225 g/8 oz dried split green peas

100 g/4 oz smoked sausage

1 leek (white parts only), sliced

1 celery stick, sliced

1 carrot, sliced

50 g/2 oz celeriac, cubed

1 large tomato, chopped

1 garlic clove, crushed

1 tsp dried thyme

1 bay leaf

salt and freshly ground black pepper, to taste

Combine all the ingredients, except the salt and pepper, in the slow cooker. Cover and cook on Low for 6–8 hours. Remove the sausage. Process the soup in a food processor or blender until smooth. Slice the sausage and stir it into the soup. Season to taste with salt and pepper.

Split-pea Soup Jardinière

This 'gardener's style' split-pea soup is flavoured the old-fashioned way with a ham bone, leek, turnip and carrot.

Serves 4

1.2 litres/2 pints water

225 g/8 oz dried split green peas

1 meaty ham bone

1 small onion, quartered

1 leek (white parts only), sliced

1 celery stick, sliced

1 carrot, sliced

1 small turnip, cubed

1 large tomato, chopped

1 garlic clove, crushed

2 whole cloves

1 tsp dried thyme

1 bay leaf

salt and freshly ground black pepper, to taste

Combine all the ingredients, except the salt and pepper, in the slow cooker. Cover and cook on Low for 6–8 hours. Remove the ham bone. Remove and shred the meat. Return the shredded meat to the soup. Discard the bones and bay leaf. Season to taste with salt and pepper.

Garlic and Rosemary Cashew Nuts V

This recipe is delicious made with any type of nut and stores well so it's worth making a large quantity. Store in an airtight container.

Serves 24

700 g/1½ lb cashew nuts

40 g/1½ oz butter or margarine, melted

1 tbsp sugar

3 tbsp dried rosemary leaves, crushed

¾ tsp cayenne pepper

½ tsp garlic powder

Heat the slow cooker on High for 15 minutes. Add the cashew nuts. Drizzle the butter or margarine over the cashew nuts and toss. Sprinkle with the combined remaining ingredients and toss. Cover and cook on Low for 2 hours, stirring every hour. Turn the heat to High. Uncover and cook for 30 minutes, stirring after 15 minutes. Turn the heat to Low to keep warm for serving or remove from the slow cooker and cool.

Garlic and Pepper Almonds V

Buttery almonds with garlic and pepper go well with drinks. Try a mixture of coarsely ground black, red and green peppercorns for a gourmet touch! Make a quantity and store in an airtight container.

Serves 24

700 g/1½ lb whole unblanched almonds
50 g/2 oz butter or margarine, melted
3 garlic cloves, crushed
2–3 tsp coarsely ground pepper

Heat the slow cooker on High for 15 minutes. Add the almonds. Drizzle the butter or margarine over the almonds and toss. Sprinkle with garlic and pepper, and toss. Cover and cook on Low for 2 hours, stirring every 30 minutes. Turn the heat to High. Uncover and cook for 30 minutes, stirring after 15 minutes. Turn the heat to Low to keep warm for serving or remove from the slow cooker and cool.

Spicy-glazed Nuts V

You can use any nuts for this recipe. Make a quantity and store in an airtight container.

Serves 24

130 g/4½ oz butter or margarine, melted
50 g/2 oz icing sugar
1 tsp ground cinnamon
1 tsp mixed spice
700 g/1½ lb mixed nuts

Heat the slow cooker on High for 15 minutes. Mix the butter or margarine, sugar and spices. Pour over the nuts in a large bowl and toss. Transfer the mixture to the slow cooker. Cover and cook on High for 30 minutes. Uncover and cook until the nuts are crisply glazed, 45–60 minutes, stirring every 20 minutes. Pour the nuts in a single layer on baking trays and cool.

Sweet Curried Soy Nuts V

Soy nuts make an unusual change, but the recipe would also work well with peanuts, walnuts, blanched almonds or pecan nuts.

Serves 24

50 g/2 oz butter or margarine, melted
700 g/1½ lb roasted soy nuts
1½ tbsp sugar
1 tbsp curry powder
salt, to taste

Heat the slow cooker on High for 15 minutes. Drizzle the butter or margarine over the soy nuts in a large bowl and toss. Sprinkle with the combined sugar and curry powder, and toss. Transfer to the slow cooker. Cover and cook on Low for 2 hours, stirring every 15 minutes. Turn the heat to High. Remove the lid and cook for 30 minutes, stirring after 15 minutes. Season to taste with salt. Turn the heat to Low to keep warm for serving or remove from the slow cooker and cool.

Sugar-glazed Five-spice Pecan Nuts V

Pecan nuts are spiced and sweetened up to make an unusual and very tasty appetiser. Make a quantity and store in an airtight container.

Serves 24

130 g/4½ oz butter or margarine, melted
50 g/2 oz icing sugar
1 tsp ground cinnamon
¾ tsp Chinese five-spice powder
700 g/1½ lb pecan nut halves

Heat the slow cooker on High for 15 minutes. Mix the butter or margarine, sugar and spices. Pour over the pecans in a large bowl and toss. Transfer the mixture to the slow cooker. Cover and cook on High for 30 minutes. Uncover and cook until the nuts are crisply glazed, 45–60 minutes, stirring every 20 minutes. Pour the pecan nuts in a single layer on baking trays and cool.

Cranberry and Nut Mix V

Nutritious nuts and dried cranberries star in this savoury-sweet snack mix. Try using blueberries instead of cranberries for a change.

Serves 8

200 g/7 oz roasted almonds
40 g/1½ oz wheat squares cereal, such as Shreddies
40 g/1½ oz mini pretzel twists
175 g/6 oz dried cranberriess
vegetable cooking spray
¾ tsp crushed dried rosemary
¾ tsp thyme leaves
garlic salt, to taste

Heat the slow cooker on High for 15 minutes. Add the almonds, cereal, pretzels and cranberries. Spray the mixture generously with cooking spray and toss. Sprinkle with the herbs and toss again. Cover and cook on Low for 2 hours, stirring every 20 minutes. Turn the heat to High. Uncover and cook for 30 minutes, stirring after 15 minutes. Season to taste with garlic salt. Turn the heat to Low to keep warm for serving or remove from the slow cooker and cool.

Snack Mix V

A great snack mix for nibbling or for sharing with a gathering of friends.

Serves 16

3 cups low-fat granola
175 g/6 oz mini pretzels
6 sesame sticks, broken into halves
500 g/18 oz mixed dried fruit, coarsely chopped
butter-flavoured cooking spray
1 tsp ground cinnamon
½ tsp freshly grated nutmeg

Heat the slow cooker on High for 15 minutes. Add the granola, pretzels, sesame sticks and dried fruit. Spray the mixture generously with cooking spray and toss. Sprinkle with the combined spices and toss. Cook, uncovered, on High for 1½ hours, stirring every 30 minutes. Keep warm on Low for serving or remove from the slow cooker and cool.

Herb Party Mix V

A colourful snack mix, with lots of variety!

Serves 16

100 g/4 oz small square cheese biscuits
130 g/4½ oz mini pretzels
1½ cups potato sticks
175 g/6 oz peanuts
100 g/4 oz butter or margarine, melted
½ tsp Tabasco sauce
1 tbsp dried Italian herb seasoning
½–1 tsp garlic salt

Heat the slow cooker on High for 15 minutes. Add the cheese biscuits, pretzels, potato sticks and peanuts. Drizzle with the combined remaining ingredients and toss. Cook, uncovered, on High for 1½ hours, stirring every 30 minutes. Keep warm on Low for serving or remove from the slow cooker and cool.

Chutney Cheese Dip V

Fruity, spicy flavours with cheese make a fun dip for crudités or pitta bread pieces.

Serves 16

450 g/1 lb soft cheese, at room temperature

225 g/8 oz Cheddar cheese, grated

150 g/5 oz chopped mango chutney

½ onion, finely chopped

40 g/1½ oz chopped raisins

2–4 tsp finely chopped fresh root ginger

2–4 garlic cloves, crushed

1–2 tsp curry powder

dippers: baked pitta bread pieces, assorted vegetables

Put the cheeses in a a 1.5 litre/2½ pint slow cooker. Cover and cook on Low until the cheese has melted, about 30 minutes. Mix in the remaining ingredients, except the dippers. Cover and cook until hot, 1–1½ hours. Serve with dippers.

Pepperoni Cheese Dip

Salami, ham, or smoked turkey can be substituted for the pepperoni in this piquant creamy dip.

Serves 10

225 g/8 oz soft cheese with onions and chives

175 g/6 oz Emmental or Gruyère cheese, grated

90 g/3½ oz sliced pepperoni, chopped

½ green pepper, chopped

¼ tsp cayenne pepper

120–150 ml/4–5 fl oz full-fat milk

dippers: assorted vegetables, crackers, breadsticks

Put the cheeses in a the slow cooker. Cover and cook on Low until the cheeses have melted, about 30 minutes. Mix in the remaining ingredients, except the dippers. Cover and cook until hot, about 1½ hours. Serve with dippers.

Hot Artichoke Dip V

A lovely creamy artichoke mixture that's given a little kick with cayenne.

Serves 16

100 g/4 oz soft cheese, at room temperature
400 g/14 oz artichoke hearts, drained and finely chopped
40 g/1½ oz freshly grated Parmesan cheese
120 ml/4 fl oz mayonnaise
120 ml/4 fl oz soured cream
1–2 tsp lemon juice
1 spring onion, thinly sliced
2 garlic cloves, crushed
salt and cayenne pepper, to taste
dippers: assorted vegetables, breadsticks, crackers

Put the soft cheese in a 1.5 litre/2½ pint slow cooker. Cover and cook on Low until the cheese has melted, about 30 minutes. Mix in the remaining ingredients, except the salt, cayenne pepper and dippers. Cover and cook until hot, 1–1½ hours. Season to taste with salt and cayenne pepper. Serve with dippers.

Curry-spiced Mixed Nuts V

This very simple blend of sweet, savoury and buttery flavours is a popular spicy nibble. Make a quantity and store in an airtight container.

Serves 24

700 g/1½ lb mixed nuts
50 g/2 oz butter or margarine, melted
2 tbsp sugar
1½ tsp curry powder
1 tsp garlic powder
1 tsp ground cinnamon

Heat the slow cooker on High for 15 minutes. Add the nuts. Drizzle the butter or margarine over the nuts and toss. Sprinkle with the combined remaining ingredients and toss. Cover and cook on Low for 2 hours, stirring every 20 minutes. Turn the heat to High. Uncover and cook for 30 minutes, stirring after 15 minutes. Turn the heat to Low to keep warm for serving or remove from the slow cooker and cool.

Spinach and Artichoke Dip V

Colourful and creamy – a great dip for parties.

Serves 16

100 g/4 oz soft cheese, at room temperature

400 g/14 oz artichoke hearts, drained and finely chopped

130 g/4½ oz well drained, thawed, frozen chopped spinach

½ roasted red pepper, chopped

40 g/1½ oz freshly grated Parmesan cheese

120 ml/4 fl oz mayonnaise

120 ml/4 fl oz soured cream

1–2 tsp lemon juice

1 spring onion, thinly sliced

2 garlic cloves, crushed

salt and cayenne pepper, to taste

dippers: assorted vegetables, breadsticks, crackers

Put the soft cheese in a 1.5 litre/2½ pint slow cooker. Cover and cook on Low until the cheese has melted, about 30 minutes. Mix in the remaining ingredients, except the salt, cayenne pepper and dippers. Cover and cook until hot, 1–1½ hours. Season to taste with salt and cayenne pepper. Serve with dippers.

Artichoke and Prawn Dip

Make sure you thaw the prawns, if frozen.

Serves 16   ·

100 g/4 oz soft cheese, at room temperature

400 g/14 oz artichoke hearts, drained and finely chopped

130 g/4½ oz well drained, thawed, frozen chopped spinach

90 g/3½ oz chopped prawns

1–2 tbsp drained capers

½ roasted red pepper, chopped

40 g/1½ oz freshly grated Parmesan cheese

120 ml/4 fl oz mayonnaise

120 ml/4 fl oz soured cream

1–2 tsp lemon juice

1 spring onion, thinly sliced

2 garlic cloves, crushed

salt and cayenne pepper, to taste

dippers: assorted vegetables, breadsticks, crackers

Put the soft cheese in a 1.5 litre/2½ pint slow cooker. Cover and cook on Low until the cheese has melted, about 30 minutes. Mix in the remaining ingredients, except the salt, cayenne pepper and dippers. Cover and cook until hot, 1–1½ hours. Season to taste with salt and cayenne pepper. Serve with dippers.

Hot Crab and Artichoke Dip

Smooth and delicious – with a hint of spice.

Serves 16

100 g/4 oz soft cheese, at room temperature

400 g/14 oz artichoke hearts, drained and finely chopped

130 g/4½ oz well drained, thawed, frozen chopped spinach

350 g/12 oz coarsely chopped white crab meat

2 tbsp chopped pickled jalapeño, or medium-hot, chilli

½ roasted red pepper, chopped

40 g/1½ oz freshly grated Parmesan cheese

120 ml/4 fl oz mayonnaise

120 ml/4 fl oz soured cream

1–2 tsp lemon juice

1 spring onion, thinly sliced

2 garlic cloves, crushed

salt and cayenne pepper, to taste

dippers: assorted vegetables, breadsticks, crackers

Put the soft cheese in a a 1.5 litre/2½ pint slow cooker. Cover and cook on Low until the cheese has melted, about 30 minutes. Mix in the remaining ingredients, except the salt, cayenne pepper and dippers. Cover and cook until hot, 1–1½ hours. Season to taste with salt and cayenne pepper. Serve with dippers.

Beef and Thousand Island Dip

This is like a combination of all the favourite sandwich fillings, but in a dip!

Serves 12

175 g/6 oz soft cheese, at room temperature

100 g/4 oz Emmental or Gruyère cheese, grated

100 g/4 oz sauerkraut, rinsed and drained

50 g/2 oz cooked beef, chopped

2 tbsp thousand island salad dressing

1 tbsp snipped fresh chives

1 tsp caraway seeds, lightly crushed

dippers: halved rye bread slices, assorted vegetables

Put the cheeses in the slow cooker. Cover and cook on Low until the cheeses have melted, about 30 minutes. Mix in the remaining ingredients, except the dippers. Cover and cook until hot, 1–1½ hours. Serve with dippers.

Dried Beef and Onion Dip

This warm, creamy dip can also be served cold – just beat soft cheese and soured cream until smooth and mix in the remaining ingredients. You can buy beef jerky in specialist outlets, but you could also make the dip with cold roast beef.

Serves 16

350 g/12 oz soft cheese, at room temperature
175 ml/6 fl oz mayonnaise
130 g/4½ oz dried beef jerky, chopped
2 spring onions, thinly sliced
2 tbsp dried onion flakes
1 tsp garlic salt
dippers: crackers, assorted vegetables, breadsticks

Put the soft cheese in the slow cooker. Cover and cook on Low until the cheese has melted, about 30 minutes. Mix in the remaining ingredients, except the dippers. Cover and cook until hot, 1–1½ hours. Serve with dippers.

Toasted Onion Dip

The flavour secret here is toasting the dried onion flakes. The dip is served hot or can be cooled to room temperature.

Serves 12

6–8 tbsp dried onion flakes
450 g/1 lb soft cheese, at room temperature
150 ml/¼ pint plain yoghurt
150 ml/¼ pint mayonnaise
4 small spring onions, chopped
3 garlic cloves, crushed
½ tsp beef bouillon granules
120–175 ml/4–6 fl oz semi-skimmed milk
1–2 tsp lemon juice
4–6 drops red pepper sauce
salt and white pepper, to taste
dippers: assorted vegetables, breadsticks

Cook the onion flakes in a small frying pan over medium to medium-low heat until toasted, 3–4 minutes, stirring frequently. Remove from the heat. Put the soft cheese in a 1.5 litre/2½ pint slow cooker. Cover and cook on Low until the cheese has melted, about 30 minutes. Mix in the yoghurt, mayonnaise, spring onions, garlic, bouillon, onion flakes and 120 ml/4 fl oz milk. Cover and cook until hot, 1–1½ hours. Season to taste with lemon juice, pepper sauce, salt and white pepper. Stir in the remaining milk, if desired for consistency. Serve with dippers.

Garlic and Three-cheese Dip V

If you like, use minced garlic from a jar to make this recipe extra-easy. You will need 2–3 tbsp. This dip can also be a spread. Beat the cheeses until blended and mix in the garlic, pepper and milk.

Serves 12

225 g/8 oz soft cheese, at room temperature
50 g/2 oz goats' cheese
25 g/1 oz freshly grated Parmesan cheese
1–2 large garlic cloves, preferably roasted, crushed
a pinch of white pepper
150 ml¼ pt semi-skimmed milk
dippers: assorted vegetables and crackers

Put the soft cheese and goats' cheese in a 1.5 litre/2½ pint slow cooker. Cover and cook on Low until the cheese has melted, about 30 minutes. Mix in the Parmesan cheese, garlic, white pepper and 120 ml/4 fl oz milk. Cover and cook until hot, 1–1½ hours. Stir in the remaining milk, if desired for consistency. Serve with dippers.

Chilli con Queso V

If you prefer a dip with less heat, substitute green peppers and 2–3 tsp minced jalapeño chillies for the poblano chillies.

Serves 12

2 small poblano or other mild chillies, halved
225 g/8 oz processed cheese slices, chopped
100 g/4 oz mature Cheddar cheese, grated
1 small onion, finely chopped
2 small tomatoes, finely chopped
½ tsp dried oregano
2–4 tbsp semi-skimmed milk
tortilla chips

Put the chillies, skin sides up, on a baking tray. Bake at 220ºC/gas 7/fan oven 200ºC until the chillies are browned and soft, about 20 minutes. Cool. Discard the seeds and stems, and chop coarsely.

Put the cheeses in a 1.5 litre/2½ pint slow cooker. Cover and cook on Low until the cheeses have melted, about 30 minutes. Add the chillies and the remaining ingredients, except the tortilla chips. Cover and cook until hot, 1–1½ hours. Serve with tortilla chips.

Black Bean and Green Chilli with Cheese V

This dip is fiery! Reduce the amount of crushed chilli flakes and/or omit the red pepper sauce for a milder dip.

Serves 16

225 g/8 oz Monterey Jack or Cheddar cheese, cubed
225 g/8 oz soft cheese, at room temperature
250 ml/8 fl oz mayonnaise
50 g/2 oz freshly grated Parmesan cheese
90 g/3½ oz drained, canned black or red kidney beans, rinsed
100 g/4 oz green chillies from a jar, diced
2 garlic cloves, crushed
2 tsp crushed chilli flakes
½–1 tsp red pepper sauce
dippers: tortilla chips, assorted vegetables

Put the Monterey Jack or Cheddar cheese and soft cheese in a 1.5 litre/2½ pint slow cooker. Cover and cook on Low until the cheeses have melted, about 30 minutes. Mix in the remaining ingredients, except the dippers. Cover and cook until hot, 1–1½ hours. Serve with dippers.

Black Bean and Chorizo with Cheese

Milder but still really tasty.

Serves 16

225 g/8 oz Monterey Jack or Cheddar cheese, cubed

225 g/8 oz soft cheese, at room temperature

¼ recipe Mexican Chorizo

250 ml/8 fl oz mayonnaise

1–2 tsp pickled jalapeño or other medium-hot chillies

50 g/2 oz freshly grated Parmesan cheese

90 g/3½ oz drained, canned black or red kidney beans, rinsed

2 garlic cloves, crushed

dippers: tortilla chips, assorted vegetables

Put the Monterey Jack or Cheddar cheese and soft cheese in a 1.5 litre/2½ pint slow cooker. Cover and cook on Low until the cheeses have melted, about 30 minutes. Mix in the remaining ingredients, except the dippers. Cover and cook until hot, 1–1½ hours. Serve with dippers.

Queso Wraps

The Mexican Chorizo can be used in many Mexican recipes. For the best flavour, make it several hours in advance and refrigerate, so that the flavours meld.

Serves 16

175 g/6 oz Cheddar cheese, grated
100 g/4 oz processed cheese, cubed
½ roasted red pepper from a jar, chopped
120–175 ml/4–6 fl oz semi-skimmed milk
¼ quantity Mexican Chorizo
16 flour or corn tortilla wraps (15 cm/6 in), warmed
thinly sliced spring onion and chopped fresh coriander, to garnish

Put the cheeses in a 1.5 litre/2½ pint slow cooker. Cover and cook on Low until the cheeses have melted, about 30 minutes. Mix in the remaining ingredients, except the tortillas and garnishes. Cover and cook until hot, 1–1½ hours. Spoon about 3 tbsp of the cheese mixture into the centre of each wrap. Sprinkle with spring onion and fresh coriander, and roll up.

Refried Bean Dip V

Refried black beans can also be used in this Mexican dip.

Serves 16

225 g/8 oz processed cheese, cubed
2 x 400 g/14 oz cans refried beans
50 ml/2 fl oz taco sauce or salsa
3 spring onions, chopped
1–2 tbsp chopped pickled jalapeño or other medium-hot chillies
dippers: tortilla chips, assorted vegetables

Put the cheese in a 1.5 litre/2½ pint slow cooker. Cover and cook on Low until the cheese has melted, about 30 minutes. Mix in the remaining ingredients, except the dippers. Cover and cook until hot, 1–1½ hours. Serve with dippers.

Spicy Cheese and Seafood Dip

Plenty of ground pepper adds a definite hot accent to this very easy
dip of cheese, prawns and crab meat.

Serves 8

225 g/8 oz Monterey Jack or mature Cheddar cheese, cubed
225 g/8 oz soft cheese, at room temperature
freshly grated black pepper
175 ml/6 fl oz full-fat milk
175 g/6 oz cooked prawns, thawed if frozen, chopped
175 g/6 oz white crab meat
50 g/2 oz pitted green olives, chopped
dippers: assorted vegetables, crackers, breadsticks

Put the cheeses in a 1.5 litre/2½ pint slow cooker. Cover and cook
on Low until the cheese has melted, about 30 minutes. Add plenty
of black pepper. Mix in the remaining ingredients, except the
dippers. Cover and cook until hot, 1–1½ hours. Serve with dippers.

Easy Monterey Jack Prawn Dip

Use half Cheddar and half Monterey Jack, if you like.

Serves 8

450 g/1 lb Monterey Jack or mature Cheddar cheese, cubed
225 g/8 oz soft cheese, at room temperature
freshly grated black pepper
175 ml/6 fl oz full-fat milk
350 g/12 oz cooked prawns, thawed if frozen, chopped
50 g/2 oz pitted black olives, chopped
dippers: assorted vegetables, crackers, breadsticks

Put the cheeses in a 1.5 litre/2½ pint slow cooker. Cover and cook on Low until the cheese has melted, about 30 minutes. Add plenty of black pepper. Mix in the remaining ingredients, except the dippers. Cover and cook until hot, 1–1½ hours. Serve with dippers.

Smoked Salmon Dip

Not just any smoked salmon dip, this version has artichoke hearts, capers and garlic for a dip with zip! Any smoked fish can be substituted for the salmon, if you like.

Serves 16

225 g/8 oz reduced-fat soft cheese, at room temperature
375 ml/13 fl oz mayonnaise
400 g/14 oz can artichoke hearts, drained and chopped
350 g/12 oz smoked salmon
50 g/2 oz freshly grated Parmesan cheese
40 g/1½ oz drained capers
3 large garlic cloves, crushed
3–4 dashes Tabasco sauce
dippers: assorted vegetables, crackers

Put the soft cheese in a 1.5 litre/2½ pint slow cooker. Cover and cook on Low until the cheese has melted, about 30 minutes. Mix in the remaining ingredients, except the dippers. Cover and cook until hot, 1–1½ hours. Serve with dippers.

Smoked Mackerel Dip

A simple and tasty option.

Serves 16

225 g/8 oz reduced-fat goats' cheese
175 ml/6 fl oz soured cream
175 ml/6 fl oz mayonnaise
350 g/12 oz smoked mackerel
50 g/2 oz freshly grated Parmesan cheese
40 g/1½ oz drained capers
3 large garlic cloves, crushed
3–4 dashes Tabasco sauce
dippers: assorted vegetables, crackers

Put the soft cheese in a 1.5 litre/2½ pint slow cooker. Cover and cook on Low until the cheese has melted, about 30 minutes. Mix in the remaining ingredients, except the dippers. Cover and cook until hot, 1–1½ hours. Serve with dippers.

Aubergine Caviar V

Tenderly cooked aubergine makes a lovely smooth base for a dip with garlic, yoghurt and oregano.

Serves 6

1 large aubergine (about 700 g/1½ lb)
2 tomatoes, finely chopped
½ onion, finely chopped
50 ml/2 fl oz yoghurt
3 garlic cloves, crushed
2 tbsp olive oil
½ tsp dried oregano
1–2 tbsp lemon juice
salt and freshly ground black pepper, to taste
dippers: pitta bread wedges

Pierce the aubergine in several places with a fork and put in the slow cooker. Cover and cook on Low until tender, 4–5 hours. Cool to room temperature.

Cut the aubergine in half. Scoop out the pulp with a spoon. Mash the aubergine and mix with the remaining ingredients, seasoning to taste with lemon juice, salt and pepper. Serve with dippers.